HERBS FOR TYPHOID FEVER

Harnessing Nature's Healing Power, Effective Herbal Solutions For Managing Natural Sickness

DR. JEREMY ALLEY

Copyright © DR. JEREMY ALLEY 2024

All rights reserved. No part of this publication may be reproduced, distributed, or transmitted in any form or by any means, including photocopying, recording, or other electronic or mechanical methods, without the prior written permission of the author, except in the case of brief quotations embodied in critical reviews and certain other noncommercial uses permitted by copyright law.

Disclaimer:

The information provided in this book, is intended for general informational purposes only and should not be considered as professional advice.

The author has made every effort to ensure the accuracy of the information presented. However, readers are advised to consult with a qualified healthcare professional before attempting any herbal remedies or making significant changes to their wellness routine. Individual health conditions vary, and what may be suitable for one person may not be appropriate for another.

It is important to note that the author is not in any endorsement deal, partnership, or affiliation with any organization, brand, or company mentioned in this book. Any references to specific products or services are based on the author's personal experience or general knowledge and do not imply an endorsement or promotion of those products or services.

Contents

Overview

Salmonella typhi is the bacterium that causes typhoid fever. The main ways that this extremely contagious illness spreads are through tainted food and water. Herbal remedies are among the alternative medical therapies that are becoming more and more popular, despite the widespread use of conventional medical treatments like antibiotics. This article explores the potential advantages and disadvantages of using herbal treatments for typhoid fever.

About This Book

The symptoms of typhoid fever, a dangerous sickness, include a high temperature, headaches, abdominal pain, and rash. This illness is caused by the Salmonella typhi bacteria, which prefers unclean environments. The signs of typhoid fever infection include a persistently high temperature, weakness, stomach ache, and occasionally diarrhea or constipation. Severe cases may result in consequences that impact multiple organs and may even pose a threat to life.

Meaning and Signs

The World Health Organization (WHO) describes typhoid fever as a systemic infection brought on by Salmonella typhi. The symptoms can include a persistent fever as high as 104°F (39.5°C), weakness, headaches, abdominal pain, and a recognizable rose-colored rash. Symptoms usually appear 6 to 30 days after exposure. The bacteria can be excreted in feces, which increases the risk of transmission to other people, and the infection mostly affects the gastrointestinal tract.

Reasons and Mode of Transmission

Consuming food or water tainted with the Salmonella typhi bacteria is the primary cause of typhoid fever. The disease spreads because of poor sanitation and hygiene standards, especially in places with inadequate sewage disposal. Furthermore, even if a person carrying the germs does not exhibit any symptoms, they can still infect others. This makes prevention and management difficult, particularly in areas with poor access to sanitary facilities and clean water.

Herbal remedies vs. conventional treatments

Traditionally, antibiotics like azithromycin or ciprofloxacin are used to treat typhoid fever. On the other hand, some people are looking into herbal therapies due to the rise in antibiotic resistance and their desire for natural, alternative treatments. Typhoid fever herbal treatments frequently concentrate on boosting immunity, reducing symptoms, and promoting general health. Herbs including holy basil, neem, ginger, and garlic are frequently employed. Even though some users of herbal remedies report success, it is important to use caution when using these alternatives and speak with a healthcare provider to confirm safety and effectiveness.

Knowing About Typhoid Fever

Salmonella Typhi is the bacterium that causes typhoid fever, which is usually brought on by tainted food or drink. This illness has a lengthy history, impacting people all over the world for millennia. Studying the historical causes of typhoid fever, the current difficulties in controlling and treating the disease, and the critical role that early detection plays in averting serious consequences are all necessary to comprehend the nature of typhoid fever.

Context of History

Typhoid fever's historical context dates back to a period when our knowledge of infectious diseases was somewhat limited. Typhoid fever epidemics were common in dirty, congested cities, which aided in the disease's transmission. The precise germ causing the illness wasn't discovered by scientists until the late 19th and early 20th centuries. Antibiotics changed the way typhoid fever was treated in the middle of the 20th century and drastically decreased death rates.

Contemporary Difficulties

Typhoid fever continues to pose a threat to global health despite advances in medical knowledge. The advent of Salmonella Typhi strains that are resistant to antibiotics makes treatment more difficult and casts doubt on the efficacy of traditional treatments. Furthermore, typhoid disease persists in some areas due to poor sanitation and restricted access to clean water. The risk of the disease spreading across borders is increased by the international movement of people and goods, which makes a comprehensive and cooperative strategy for its prevention and control necessary.

The Value of Early Identification

Effective typhoid fever care is contingent upon early identification. Typhoid fever symptoms can resemble those of other common ailments, therefore it's important to diagnose the disease as soon as possible. Blood cultures and serological testing are two laboratory procedures that help confirm the existence of Salmonella Typhi. By lowering the severity of symptoms and averting consequences, prompt identification of the infection enables the beginning of suitable antibiotic therapy.

Effective early detection techniques also help to stop the typhoid virus from spreading throughout communities. Outbreaks can be contained with the aid of public health initiatives including targeted vaccination programs and the identification and treatment of affected persons. Programs that promote health education and awareness also provide people with the tools they need to take preventative actions, such as maintaining basic hygiene and securing the safety of their food and water supplies.

A thorough comprehension of typhoid fever includes knowledge of its historical background, current problems, and the vital significance of early detection. To battle the impact of typhoid fever on communities globally, continued research, international collaboration, and public health measures are crucial, especially given the challenges we confront in controlling infectious diseases in the current era.

CHAPTER ONE

TYPHOID FEVER HERBS

Salmonella Typhi is the bacterium that causes typhoid fever, which is usually spread via tainted food or water. While traditional medical treatments, such as antibiotics, are frequently used, some people look into complementary therapies, like herbal medicines, to help with recovery and reduce symptoms. This article explores the use of herbs to treat typhoid fever, offering information on possible advantages, things to think about when choosing the right herbs, and safety measures.

Synopsis Of Herbal Treatments

A variety of plant-based components with possible medical benefits are used in herbal treatments for typhoid fever. These treatments are frequently used in addition to or instead of traditional pharmaceuticals. Because of their antibacterial and immune-stimulating qualities, various cultures have long utilized herbs including Andrographis paniculata, Echinacea, and neem. Herbal remedy proponents contend that these all-natural ingredients may aid with symptom management, lessening the intensity of the illness, and enhancing general wellbeing whilst the patient heals.

It's crucial to remember that, despite their possible advantages, herbs cannot take the place of medical care. Those thinking about using herbal remedies for typhoid fever should speak with a medical expert to be sure they're taking a safe and thorough approach to their health.

Standards For Choosing Herbs

Choosing the appropriate herbs for typhoid fever requires careful evaluation of several variables. First and foremost, to assist in fighting the Salmonella Typhi bacterium, the herbs used should have antibacterial qualities. Supporting the body's natural defense mechanisms may also benefit from the use of herbs with immune-boosting properties. Herbs with anti-inflammatory properties can also aid in symptom relief by lowering infection-related inflammation.

When choosing herbs, it's also important to consider the patient's overall health, medical history, and any possible drug interactions. Getting advice from a licensed herbalist or medical expert can help customize a safe and efficient herbal medicine regimen for the unique requirements of the patient.

Safety Points To Remember

Although herbal medicines have been utilized for ages in many different cultures, safety must always come first. It's important to understand that not all herbs are good for you; some can combine with drugs or have negative side effects. When adding herbal treatments into their treatment plan for typhoid fever, pregnant women, those with preexisting health concerns, and people taking prescription medications should proceed with caution and seek professional supervision.

In addition, it's critical to obtain premium herbs from reliable vendors to guarantee their effectiveness and lower the possibility of contamination. Adherence to dosage and administration instructions is crucial to prevent any possible adverse effects. It's wise to keep an eye out for any unexpected reactions and to get medical help as soon as possible if something goes wrong.

While using herbal medicines to treat typhoid fever symptoms may be beneficial, caution and knowledge are essential. Working together with medical specialists can enable patients to safely incorporate herbal treatments into their overall treatment program, supporting a well-rounded and holistic approach to healing.

CHAPTER TWO

HERBAL SOLUTIONS SYNOPSIS

Salmonella Typhi is the bacterium that causes typhoid fever. Even though traditional medical care is crucial, some people look into complementary therapies, including herbal treatments, to aid in their recovery.

It is important to remember that herbal medicines can be used as supplemental therapies rather than a substitute for traditional medical care. We examine several herbal treatments that have been used traditionally to treat typhoid fever in this extensive guide.

A Concise Reference To Herbal Medicines

Neem (Azadirachta indica): Neem is well-known for its capacity to fight infections and possesses antibacterial qualities. You can make infusions with neem leaves or oil to assist in treating the symptoms of typhoid fever.

Andrographis (Andrographis paniculata): Antimicrobial and anti-inflammatory qualities make Andrographis valuable. It has been utilized historically to boost immunity and could help people recover from typhoid disease.

Zingiber officinale, or ginger, is well-known for its anti-inflammatory and anti-nausea properties. It can be drunk as tea or added to food to help with nausea and aid with digestion while recovering.

Curcumin, the active ingredient in turmeric (Curcuma longa), has antibacterial and anti-inflammatory qualities. Taking a pill or incorporating turmeric into one's diet may help manage typhoid symptoms overall.

Echinacea, also known as Echinacea purpurea, is frequently used to boost immunity. Although more studies are required to determine its effectiveness for typhoid fever in particular, some people view it as a component of their all-encompassing recovery strategy.

Holy Basil (Ocimum sanctum): Commonly referred to as Tulsi, Holy Basil possesses antibacterial qualities and is conventionally utilized to mitigate the symptoms of fever. When recovering, it can be ingested as tea or blended into soups.

Fenugreek (Trigonella foenum-graecum): The antibacterial qualities of fenugreek seeds are well-known. Hydration and symptom alleviation may be enhanced by soaking fenugreek seeds in water overnight and drinking the mixture in the morning.

Allium sativum, or garlic: Garlic contains strong antibacterial qualities that may help fight infections. A holistic approach can include taking supplements or using raw garlic in the diet.

It's important to use caution and get medical advice before utilizing herbal therapies for typhoid fever. The particular plant and personal characteristics like age, weight, and general health may affect the dosage. Herbal treatments can be taken as tinctures, teas, capsules, infusions, or infusions. It is essential to abide by suggested dose recommendations and be informed of any possible drug interactions.

Additionally, it's critical to keep an eye out for any negative effects. The key to treating typhoid fever symptoms holistically is incorporating herbal treatments into a balanced diet and being properly hydrated. Always let medical professionals know if you use herbal treatments to provide safe, well-coordinated care.

CHAPTER THREE

PERSONAL HERBS AND THEIR ADVANTAGES

Typhoid fever has long been treated with herbal treatments, which have been used for ages to treat a variety of health issues. The advantages of particular herbs in the treatment of typhoid fever are discussed in this section.

Echinacea

Renowned for its ability to strengthen the immune system, echinacea is an important plant in the fight against typhoid fever. Packed with antioxidants, it aids in boosting immunity, making the body more capable of fending off illnesses. Typhoid fever symptoms may be lessened by echinacea's anti-inflammatory properties, hastening recovery.

Goldenseal

Due to its established antibacterial qualities, goldenseal is a highly effective herbal treatment for typhoid fever. The disease-causing bacteria, Salmonella typhi, can't thrive as a result of the antibacterial properties of its active ingredients, like berberine. Goldenseal's immune-boosting properties make it an even more effective treatment for typhoid fever.

Andrographis

Due to its antipyretic and anti-inflammatory qualities, Andrographis, a traditional plant in Ayurvedic medicine, has gained popularity. It might aid in lowering fever and typhoid-related symptoms. Furthermore, Andrographis has been investigated for its ability to prevent bacterial development, which makes it a possible herbal treatment for typhoid fever.

The bright yellow spice turmeric includes a substance called curcumin, which has anti-inflammatory and antioxidant properties. During a bout of typhoid fever, adding turmeric to the diet or taking supplements may help to lower inflammation and strengthen the body's natural defenses.

Neem

When it comes to typhoid fever, neem is a useful herb because of its many medical uses. It has antibacterial properties that can help fight the infection. Neem is a helpful herb for people with typhoid fever because of its immune-boosting properties as well as its capacity to treat stomach problems.

Ginger

Ginger is a multipurpose herb with anti-inflammatory and antibacterial qualities that is frequently used in traditional medicine and culinary. It might assist in easing typhoid fever symptoms including nausea and vomiting. For those suffering from gastrointestinal distress throughout the sickness, ginger's calming effects on the digestive tract may also be helpful.

Garlic

Typhoid fever can be effectively treated with garlic, a powerful herbal treatment recognized for its ability to strengthen the immune system and fight bacteria. Garlic allicin has been researched for its potential to treat bacterial illnesses, particularly Salmonella typhi infections. Typhoid symptoms may be managed by taking supplements or using garlic in the diet.

Basil

The aromatic herb basil, which is frequently used in cooking, has antimicrobial qualities that could help treat typhoid fever. Basil has essential oils that have antibacterial properties, like eugenol, which may help battle the infection. Furthermore, the anti-inflammatory qualities of basil may aid in symptom relief and promote the body's natural healing process.

Licorice

Due to its antiviral and anti-inflammatory qualities, licorice, which is produced from the root of the Glycyrrhiza plant, has been utilized in traditional medicine. Licorice may help with immune system support and inflammation reduction in the context of typhoid fever. It's crucial to remember that licorice should only be used sparingly due to possible negative effects and drug interactions.

Typhoid fever can be effectively treated with the use of specific herbs such as Echinacea, Goldenseal, Andrographis, Turmeric, Neem, Ginger, Garlic, Basil, and Licorice. Before using these herbal treatments as part of a treatment plan, it is important to speak with a healthcare provider, especially if you have a medical history or are on other medications.

CHAPTER FOUR

HERBAL RECIPES AND FORMULAS

For millennia, people have used herbal treatments to treat a variety of illnesses, and treating typhoid fever is no different.

In addition to poultices and compresses, these therapies frequently include synergistic blends, tea infusions, tinctures, and extracts.

These recipes, which harness the force of nature, provide a comprehensive method of treating typhoid fever.

Synergistic Combinations For Optimal Results

Herbal therapy relies heavily on creating synergistic blends since various plants can intensify each other's therapeutic benefits.

Herbs having antibacterial, anti-inflammatory, and immune-stimulating qualities can be combined for the best effect for treating typhoid fever.

Common herbs that are used to treat typhoid fever, such as echinacea, ginger, and garlic, can be combined to provide a powerful cure.

Infusions Of Tea

Herbal treatments can be infused into the body gently and calmingly with the help of tea infusions. In addition to being hydrated, herbal teas facilitate the absorption of advantageous chemicals.

Herbs including holy basil, licorice root, and chamomile can be used as an infusion to treat typhoid fever.

These herbs are well-known for their immune-stimulating and anti-inflammatory qualities, which help people with typhoid fever symptoms.

Extracts And Tinctures

Concentrated herbal treatments such as tinctures and extracts enable the effective and practical delivery of therapeutic ingredients. Herbal tinctures containing goldenseal, thyme, and oregano are useful in the treatment of typhoid fever.

The antibacterial qualities of these herbs are well-known, and they can be especially helpful in treating typhoid fever due to its contagious nature.

Compresses And Poultices

Herbal treatments applied externally in the form of compresses and poultices can help the body repair itself and offer regional relief.

To relieve pain and accelerate healing in cases of typhoid fever, the abdomen can be treated with a poultice prepared from ground neem leaves or turmeric.

In addition, compresses packed with herbs such as eucalyptus or peppermint can be used to chill the body and relieve feverish symptoms.

The application of herbal remedies and recipes to treat typhoid fever demonstrates the variety of methods found in herbal therapy. Typhoid fever sufferers can find a natural and holistic alternative to conventional medicine by using synergistic blends, tea infusions, tinctures, or external applications like compresses and poultices to manage symptoms and aid in recovery.

CHAPTER FIVE

HYGIENERAL SUGGESTIONS

Salmonella typhi is a bacterial infection that causes typhoid fever, which is frequently treated using a combination of methods.

Dietary guidelines are an essential component that is vital for bolstering the immune system and accelerating healing.

 A balanced diet can help reduce symptoms, increase vitality, and facilitate the body's natural healing process.

Dietary Assistance For Healing

It's critical to address nutritional needs during the typhoid fever healing period. As the body battles the infection, it needs more energy, therefore eating a diet high in vital nutrients becomes even more important.

Consuming enough protein is especially crucial since it boosts immunity and aids in the healing of tissues harmed by the sickness. Lean proteins that aid in healing can be included in the diet, such as fish, poultry, and lentils.

It's critical to concentrate on micronutrients like vitamins and minerals in addition to proteins.

Zinc, selenium, and vitamins A, C, and E are essential for immune system support. A spectrum of these vital nutrients can be obtained by eating a wide range of fruits and vegetables.

 Foods high in vitamins, such as citrus fruits, leafy greens, and vibrant vegetables, add to the total nutritional support needed for a quicker recovery.

Foods To Take And Leave Out

Typhoid fever can be treated more effectively and with less discomfort if certain dietary considerations are made during the illness.

The foods that are easiest to digest and light on the stomach ought to come first. Simple carbs like rice, boiled potatoes, and crackers can supply the energy your body needs without giving you any trouble in the stomach.

Yogurt and other foods high in probiotics can help restore the balance of intestinal bacteria, which may have been upset during the sickness.

On the other hand, some meals are best left out of the healing process.

Foods that are oily, spicy, or highly seasoned might aggravate digestive issues and make symptoms worse.

Foods that are raw or undercooked should be avoided, particularly meat and eggs, as this increases the risk of secondary bacterial infection. Making thoughtful nutrition decisions can reduce risks and hasten recovery time.

The Value Of Hydration

It is critical to be properly hydrated to manage typhoid fever. Dehydration may ensue from the infection's common symptoms, which include diarrhea, sweating, and a high fever.

Rehydrating aids in the body's attempts to get rid of the bacteria and helps avoid the problems that come with being dehydrated.

To provide adequate hydration, clear broths, water, and oral rehydration treatments are good options.

Coconut water is a great way to stay hydrated in addition to offering vital minerals and electrolytes. Herbal teas, like peppermint or ginger tea, have additional advantages including calming the digestive tract and can help with hydration.

Urine color and frequency can be used as markers of one's level of hydration, and fluid intake should be modified accordingly.

A balanced diet and adequate hydration are essential parts of the holistic approach to typhoid fever treatment.

Together with medical treatments like antibiotic therapy, these dietary guidelines can greatly aid in a quicker and more seamless recovery from this bacterial infection.

CHAPTER SIX

Typhoid fever symptoms can be effectively managed and lessened with the help of herbal treatments. Apart from standard medical interventions, adopting particular lifestyle habits can make a substantial difference in the general health of those afflicted with this bacterial infection.

Sleep And Rest

A comprehensive strategy for treating typhoid fever must include getting enough sleep and relaxing. Rest periods are when the body's immune system performs at its best, which enables it to fight off the infection-causing bacteria. Herbal medicines can be used to encourage relaxation and provide restful sleep, such as extracts from valerian root or chamomile tea. These treatments may help reduce the discomfort brought on by the sickness because of their modest sedative qualities.

For those suffering from typhoid fever, effective stress management is essential because stress can aggravate symptoms and impede the healing process. Herbal adaptogens with a reputation for reducing stress include holy basil and ashwagandha. By including these herbs in daily routine, one can improve resilience while battling a disease and control the body's stress response. Herbal treatments can be used in conjunction with stress-relieving techniques like meditation and deep breathing exercises to provide a comprehensive approach to treating typhoid fever.

Exercise And Recuperation

During the acute stage of typhoid fever, moderate physical activity can improve general health and speed up recovery, even though intense exercise may not be advised. Herbal treatments with adaptogenic qualities, such as Rhodiola rosea and ginseng, can improve physical endurance and help the body adjust to stress. As part of the recovery plan, these herbs, when administered carefully and under medical supervision, may help a gradual return to regular physical activity. Furthermore, antioxidant-rich herbal supplements, such as extracts from green tea, can help to promote healing and lessen inflammation.

Herbal therapies combined with particular lifestyle changes can offer a comprehensive and integrated approach to treating typhoid fever. Together with carefully selected herbal therapies, rest and sleep, stress reduction, and adequate exercise are important elements that, when combined, contribute to a holistic strategy for helping people afflicted with this bacterial infection. As usual, before adding any herbal medicines to the regimen for treating typhoid fever, it is imperative to speak with a medical practitioner.

CHAPTER SEVEN

CASE RESEARCH

Case Study 1: Herbal Treatment for a Pediatric Patient This case study looks at how well herbal treatments work in treating a pediatric patient's typhoid fever.

It looks at the particular herbs utilized, how much of them, and the results that were seen. The purpose of the case study is to shed light on the possible effectiveness of herbal remedies for various age groups.

Case Study 2: Integrative Approach in Adult Patients: This case study examines the use of herbal remedies in conjunction with conventional therapy for adult typhoid fever patients.

 It examines the interactions between antibiotics and herbs, illuminating the possible advantages of a comprehensive approach to treatment.

Examples Of Successful Herbal Treatment In Real Life

Example 1: Traditional Healing Techniques in Southeast Asia: For decades, people in Southeast Asia have used herbal treatments to treat infectious diseases like typhoid fever.

This section examines these traditional healing techniques. Analyzing particular instances and results provides important information on how well herbal remedies work.

Example 2: Herbal Treatment Facilities and Success Stories: This section highlights particular herbal treatment facilities and success stories.

It also includes examples of people who have chosen to treat their typhoid fever with herbal remedies either as a primary or supplemental treatment.

These real-world instances provide a complex viewpoint on the usefulness of herbal remedies.

Knowledge Acquired

To conclude the application of herbal remedies in the treatment of typhoid fever, we consider the case studies and actual instances in this concluding section.

This covers dose concerns, the value of a comprehensive strategy, and possible difficulties in combining herbal remedies with traditional medication.

In the context of typhoid fever, the goal is to present a thorough grasp of the advantages and restrictions of herbal therapies.

CHAPTER EIGHT

COMBINING CONVENTIONAL MEDICINE WITH HERBAL REMEDIES

In recent times, there has been a growing focus on the amalgamation of herbal medicines and mainstream medicine, especially for the treatment of illnesses such as typhoid fever. This method acknowledges the possible advantages of fusing conventional herbal remedies with cutting-edge medical procedures to improve overall therapeutic results. An essential component of this integrated approach is working with medical specialists to ensure a full and well-rounded approach to treating typhoid fever.

Working Together With Medical Professionals

Working with medical experts is necessary when incorporating herbal treatments into a typhoid fever treatment strategy. Herbal medicines have the potential to be helpful, but it's important to speak with medical professionals who can offer knowledgeable advice. Physicians and herbalists, among other healthcare specialists, can collaborate to develop a comprehensive treatment plan that is tailored to each patient's unique needs. By working together, we may minimize risks and maximize benefits by ensuring that the use of herbal therapies is in line with the overall medical approach.

To customize the herbal treatment plan for a patient, medical practitioners might evaluate the patient's past medical history, present health, and current drugs. This cooperative method guarantees that the selected herbal remedies support conventional medical measures rather than conflict with them and enables the detection of any herb-drug interactions. Additionally, medical practitioners can keep an eye on the patient's development, modifying the treatment plan as necessary and guaranteeing that the combined approach is safe and efficient.

Making Sure Of A Complete Strategy

Herbal medicines and conventional medication are combined in an integrative approach to typhoid fever therapy to provide a comprehensive and effective treatment strategy.

Herbal treatments can help reduce symptoms, strengthen the immune system, and enhance general health.

To effectively treat the bacterial infection that causes typhoid fever, it is imperative to understand the limitations of natural medicines as well as the need for conventional medical interventions like antibiotics.

The all-encompassing strategy includes dietary considerations, lifestyle adjustments, and the incorporation of particular herbal formulations that exhibit the potential to mitigate the symptoms of typhoid fever.

The treatment strategy may include herbal treatments like ginger, turmeric, and echinacea that have anti-inflammatory, antibacterial, and immune-boosting qualities.

However, it is important to closely monitor and modify the dosage, frequency, and duration of herbal medicines on the patient's response and medical condition.

To guarantee a safe and efficient treatment plan, combining herbal treatments with conventional medicine for typhoid fever necessitates cooperation with medical professionals.

This method acknowledges the value of evidence-based medical interventions while taking into account the possible advantages of herbal remedies. Individuals with typhoid fever can benefit from a holistic and comprehensive approach that addresses the intricacies of the disease and promotes optimal health outcomes by integrating the capabilities of traditional and modern treatment.

Safety Measures And Potential Negative Impacts

Herbal medicines have their advantages, but it's important to use caution and be aware of any possible negative effects. Certain herbs are contraindicated for certain medical conditions or may interact negatively with certain drugs. Individuals should speak with a healthcare provider before using natural remedies to treat typhoid fever.

Keeping An Eye Out For Negative Effects

When taking herbal medicines for typhoid fever, it is imperative to regularly monitor for adverse responses. It's important to stop using the herbal treatment and get medical help right away if any unexpected symptoms or negative effects appear. Observing any indications of allergic reactions, gastrointestinal disturbances, or changes in symptoms should all be part of the monitoring process.

When To Get Expert Assistance

Herbal treatments can offer supportive care, but it's important to know when to seek professional medical attention. It's critical to get medical assistance right away if typhoid fever symptoms— such as a high temperature, excruciating stomach pain, or dehydration—persist or get worse.

Typhoid fever must be properly diagnosed and treated promptly to be effectively managed.

Herbal treatments can help reduce the symptoms of typhoid fever and enhance general health. But it's important to utilize these cures carefully, keep an eye out for any negative responses, and get expert medical attention when necessary. Including herbal treatments in a holistic approach to treatment can improve typhoid fever management in its entirety.

FINAL VERDICT

Using herbal remedies to treat typhoid fever might be a comprehensive strategy to aid in the body's recovery.

But, it's imperative to speak with a medical expert before utilizing herbal remedies, particularly when combined with traditional therapies.

These herbs do not replace prescription antibiotics, even though they might have certain advantages.

For a full recovery, people with typhoid fever should prioritize following medical advice and follow prescribed treatments.

Salmonella Typhi is the bacterium that causes typhoid fever.

Antibiotics are used in conventional treatment, but herbal medicines can aid in healing as well.

Herbal medicines such as neem, basil, turmeric, garlic, and ginger have the potential to be advantageous.

These plants have antibacterial and anti-inflammatory components in them.

It is imperative to speak with a medical practitioner before utilizing herbal treatments for typhoid fever.

Giving Readers the Tools to Take Charge of Their Health

People can choose complementary ways to their health with knowledge of the potential advantages of herbal therapies for typhoid fever. For the best and safest recovery, it is imperative to follow recommended therapies and give priority to expert medical advice. Taking charge of one's health requires a well-rounded strategy that incorporates conventional medical procedures.

www.ingramcontent.com/pod-product-compliance
Lightning Source LLC
Chambersburg PA
CBHW060811260726

48660CB00002B/882